0

I dedicate this book to my loyal &
inspirational clients.


Challenge your limits – Don't limit your challenges!

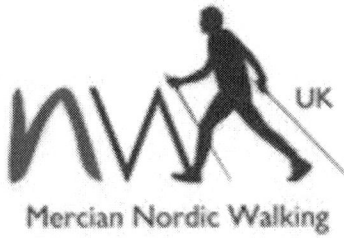

Mercian Nordic Walking

"Having had a few injuries over the last few years, training with Ian has certainly helped me to get my mojo back. My fitness has improved dramatically, allowing me to take on and win a nordic walking marathon and a 24 hour walking race. I have entered several 10k races as a Nordic walker using Ian's 10k programme as my guide. I really enjoy my training and Ian is a great coach and motivator"

- Tracey L

"Over the last 12 months training with Ian I have improved my fitness level so much that at 64 I have entered two 10k races and completed the Race to the Stones 50k in 9 hours. Thank you Ian for your help, encouragement and support. I never thought any of this was possible but it goes to show that with a good training programme anything is possible".

- Carol G

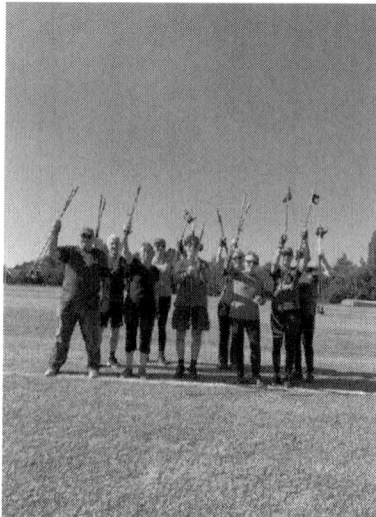

# Disclaimer:

*The author accepts no responsibility whatsoever for any injury, damage harm, illness or any negative health consequence which may occur as direct or indirect use of this material.*

*This work is for information purposes only and you must take full responsibility for the use of the material.*

*Ian Northcott BEM and Mercian Nordic Walking Limited strongly recommends that you consult with your GP or medical professional before beginning any exercise programme.*

*You should ensure that you are physically fit enough to be able to participate in the programme.*

*If you do not then please STOP reading now and do not take part in the programme.*

*Ian Northcott BEM is NOT a licenced medical care provider and has no expertise in diagnosing or treating medical conditions of any kind.*

*You must understand that when participating in any exercise or exercise programme that there is a possibility of physical injury and assume all risk yourself.*

*By reading on you accept the terms of this disclaimer.*

*For further information please visit the NHS website for information on physical activity guidelines*

# Preparing to Nordic Walk a 10km Race

### Ian Northcott BEM

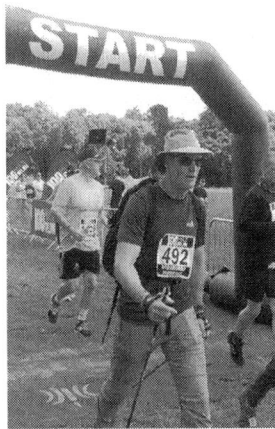

### Published by:
### Mercian Nordic Walking Limited
### 2019

# Contents

- ➢ Introduction
- ➢ Practical Considerations
- ➢ Aim of the 8 Week Programme
- ➢ Chief Medical Officer Guidelines
- ➢ FITT
- ➢ RPE
- ➢ Warm up & Cool Down/Stretches
- ➢ Nutrition
- ➢ Sessions Explained
- ➢ Week 1
- ➢ Week 2
- ➢ Week 3
- ➢ Week 4
- ➢ Week 5
- ➢ Week 6
- ➢ Week 7
- ➢ Week 8
- ➢ The Race
- ➢ Final Thoughts

# Introduction

*"A ship in post is safe but that is not what ships are built for" - U.S. Navy Rear Admiral Grace Murray Hopper*

I have been a nordic walking instructor since 2015 and I am amazed at how it has attracted so many people who would not ordinarily be interested in exercise. It is something that everyone can do at some level.

I have been even more impressed that many of these people have then gone on to complete some difficult challenges and those people are my personal inspiration.

Challenges do not have to be extreme to be effective though as long as they are actually challenging you.

Some clients have completed 10K races, 24 hour races, half marathons and marathons with others managing a mile. Both are valid as long as it is a challenge.

Sadly, in the UK mainly, Nordic walking has the reputation of walking with poles for people who could not otherwise walk almost as if they have some physical disability.

This is simply not the case as nordic walking is a sport in its own right and in Europe there are speciality nordic walking events. A brief look into the history of Nordic walking will dispel this myth.

Nordic walking is walking using poles in a similar fashion to cross country skiers as they drive themselves forward, It typically uses 90% of the body's muscles as you use your upper body to propel yourself forward.

The history is interesting in that it was first used by cross country skiers from Finland in their off season training but soon developed into a recreational activity. Bearing in mind that cross country skiing is an extremely demanding physical activity you will understand why nordic walking can be very challenging.

I have hundreds of clients who range from those who only want to enjoy a sociable walk all the way to those who want to take part in marathons and extreme challenges such as The Three Peaks Challenge.

If you are interested in improving your fitness levels and to take part in possibly your first 10k race then this book is for you.

More information on nordic walking can be found at my website www.merciannordicwalking.co.uk or at the Nordic Walking UK website www.nordicwalking.co.uk.

Instructors can be found all over the UK who offer regular sessions as well as trips and short walking holidays.

If you are interested in Nordic Walking then please visit the Nordic Walking UK website above to find a local instructor.

The idea for this book came about because I was aware some of my clients booked on to a 10K race as if it was a challenge in its own right and then simply walked it. As these clients were fully capable of walking that distance anyway it made the challenge redundant as there was no time pressure. In short, a *challenge* does actually have to BE a challenge to count.

Obviously, for some walkers who cannot currently walk 6 miles then walking that distance in itself would be the challenge. Those clients may choose to use this book to help them to improve their endurance and therefore the goal will be to complete the race. That is totally fine and the book will meet this requirement but it is suggested that you speak with a fitness professional to assist.

Readers need to be aware that many 10K races have a "cut off" time of 90 minutes at which point roads are reopened and the safety marshalling is withdrawn. (Please check with the race organisers).

I feel that this is sensible time to aim for at the first attempt and from there onwards you could seek a personal best (PB).

90 minutes for a 10K race is 4 miles per hour. Yes this is quite quick but not impossible especially if you follow a training programme.

During your race you will likely see runners who have just turned up and not followed a training programme. Do not let this be you.

# Practical Considerations

When you book your place on the race please check the following with the race organisers:

- ✓ Any cut off time when marshalling and road closures end.
- ✓ They understand that you will be walking with poles and will likely have a separate place for you to start from which is usually at the back of the group.
- ✓ Make sure that your trainers fit properly – consider having them fitted by a specialist footwear company.
- ✓ If you have not been trained in how to nordic walk then please contact Nordic Walking UK to find an instructor near you. It is imperative that you know how to use the poles properly so that you remain safe but also so that you get the maximum benefit from using them.
- ✓ Make sure you wear reflective clothing.
- ✓ Find out your race date and start the programme 8 weeks beforehand.
- ✓ Commit to the programme.

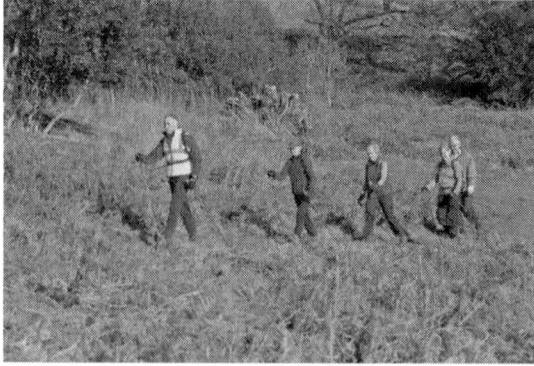

# Aim of the 8 Week Programme

The aim of this programme is to help people who are already regular Nordic walkers to prepare for a 10K event.

Participants using this programme should already be capable of walking 10km (approximately 6 miles) but now want the added challenge of completing the event in a certain time.

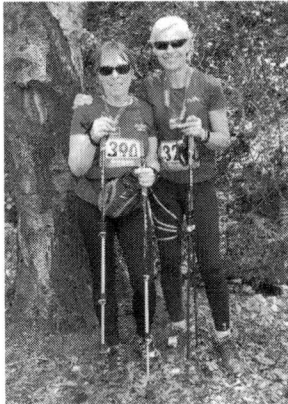

You will see that the training programme is not just walking. It involves strength sessions, cross training sessions and hill sessions.

As you progress you will realise that you will be getting fitter in many different ways and not just in your walking fitness. This is important as often people do not train all aspects of fitness.

*CV Conditioning*

*Muscle Strength & Endurance*

*Balance*

*Flexibility*

*Co-ordination*

*Stamina*

*Power*

Athletes are encouraged to keep a diary to ensure that they adhere with the programme and are encouraged to take part in group activities where possible. When clients cannot join a group session they will keep up with the programme with their own training.

It doesn't matter where you do your training but it must be safe to do so and mimic the conditions of where the race will be held (grass/tarmac etc).

Although best not to, it is acceptable to move your training days around as long as the work gets done on a week by week basis. The number of rest days must be respected.

# Chief Medical Officer Guidelines

So what are the Chief Medical Officers Guidelines for fitness and health?

Please note it is not just about how fast you can run about. Strength training is equally important and does not have to mean lifting weights.

You will notice that Mercian Nordic Walking & Outdoor Fitness offers all this and so much more.

(www.mercianoutdoorfitness.co.uk)

### Guidelines for adults aged 19 to 64

*To stay healthy, adults aged 19 to 64 should try to be **active daily** and should do:*

- *at least 150 minutes of moderate aerobic activity such as cycling or brisk walking every week **and***
- *strength exercises on 2 or more days a week that work all the major muscles (legs, hips, back, abdomen, chest, shoulders and arms)  Or:*
- *75 minutes of vigorous aerobic activity such as running or a game of singles tennis every week **and***
- *strength exercises on 2 or more days a week that work all the major muscles (legs, hips, back, abdomen, chest, shoulders and arms)  Or:*
- *a mix of moderate and vigorous aerobic activity every week – for example, 2 x 30-minute runs plus 30 minutes of brisk walking equates to 150 minutes of moderate aerobic activity **and***

> ➤ *strength exercises on 2 or more days a week that work all the major muscles (legs, hips, back, abdomen, chest, shoulders and arms)*

*A good rule is that 1 minute of vigorous activity provides the same health benefits as 2 minutes of moderate activity.*

*One way to do your recommended 150 minutes of weekly physical activity is to do 30 minutes on 5 days every week.*

*All adults should also break up long periods of sitting with light activity.*

https://www.nhs.uk/live-well/exercise/

# FITT

The FITT principle helps you to create a training programme that will help you to achieve your goals.

FITT stands for:

*Frequency*

*Intensity*

*Time*

*Type*

These are the four elements you need to manipulate if you want to improve your fitness.

If you do the same thing week in week out you will not get fitter.

If we take a beginner who has started out Nordic walking and they do a 1 mile walk at 3mph once a week.

Initially this might be enough to have a training benefit but very quickly the body becomes used to exercise. The body adapts and can then do this exercise easily and no longer goes into overload and so no training effect will take place.

This is where a lot of Mercian Nordic Walking clients remain. They are in a comfort zone and do a similar walk or activity week in week out and so will plateau.

All Mercian Nordic Walking instructors and walk leaders encourage our clients to try slightly harder sessions and also manipulate their own walks to ensure the FITT principle comes into effect.

> Frequency - If they walked their 1 mile at 3mph but increased the frequency to 3 times a week this will make them fitter.
> Intensity - If they still only walked 1 mile once a week but increased the intensity to 4mph this would make them fitter.
> Time - If they only walked once a week at 3mph but walked for 3 hours this would improve their fitness.
> Type – Instead of walking the client might try an indoor circuit training sessions or trek fit class. This would improve their fitness.

Sadly, as their body gets used to the "new" regime they will need to manipulate the FITT principle again to continue the process.

You will notice that this programme uses the FITT principle to help you prepare for your 10K race.

The programme includes:

> *CV Conditioning*
> *Cross Training*
> *Hill Sessions*
> *Rest Days*

# RPE

The RPE is the Rate of Perceived Exertion and this is how you perceive how hard you are working.

The programme gives a suggested RPE for you to work towards.

## RPE Scale

**Rate of Perceived Exertion**

| | |
|---|---|
| 10 | **Maximum Effort** <br> feels almost impossible to continue <br> no conversation possible |
| 9 | **Very Hard** <br> difficult to maintain exercise intensity <br> conversation becomes difficult |
| 7-8 | **Vigorous** <br> on the verge of becoming uncomfortable <br> breathing heavily but still able to speak |
| 4-6 | **Moderate** <br> feels like you can maintain activity for hours <br> breathing heavily but can carry on a conversation |
| 2-3 | **Light** <br> feels like you can maintain activity for hours <br> easy to breathe and carry on a conversation |
| 1 | **Very Light** <br> little to no activity |

# Warm up & Cool Down/Stretches

**WARM UP**

A warm up is to be completed as part of every session.

**Walking Element Warm Up**

Participants will walk at slow speed (RPE 3/4) for 400m of the track or equivalent distance on the trail.

Following the first 400m at slow speed then participants will slowly increase their speed up to RPE 4/5 for the second 400m.

Dynamic stretches will be completed with the following:

Hamstrings/Calves/Quads/Hip
Flexors/Shoulders/Arms/Back

**Cross Training Warm Up**

As per the walking element warm up but with lunge walks/side squats/knee hugs/half squats/chest presses using the walking poles/Lat pull downs using the walking poles

**COOL DOWN**

After every session the participants will complete a 400m walk at RPE 4 intensity and then slow down to an easy paced (RPE 2/3) for 400m. After this there will be a full body static stretch section where stretches will be held for 20-30 seconds.

A full body stretch routine that shows examples of stretches can be found here:

https://www.youtube.com/watch?v=5oj9-4ZQes4

Stretches should include:

Gastrocnemius (Calves)

Soleus (Calves)

Hamstrings (Back of upper legs)

Quads (Thighs)

Glutes (Bottom)

Hip Flexor

Shoulder

Back

Chest

Forearms

# Nutrition

This guide is not intended to give you nutrition advice and instead suggests you visit this website:

https://www.nhs.uk/live-well/eat-well/

*You cannot out-train a bad diet!*

*You cannot out-run a Mars bar!*

You might like to try out "Glow" - a healthy eating plan that can be accessed via www.mercianoutdoorfitness.co.uk.

Alcohol should be avoided.

# SESSIONS EXPLAINED

## BASELINE TESTING

This will take place on the track facility or a pre-set route.  It will contain the following:

*1600m Time Trial (Ideally 4 x 400m around athletics track)*

*Walk Lunges in 1 minute*

These tests will test the muscles used in Nordic walking.

Please contact a fitness professional if you do not know how to do these exercises or need help completing the tests.

## MODERATE WALK

An easy walk over country lanes, tracks and canal towpaths.  Clients should attain level 4-6 of the RPE for this session.

## CV CONDITIONING WALKS

These are harder sessions where you will be pushing yourselves a little bit harder up to RPE level 7 or 8 for a shorter distance within a longer walk.

*1km Moderate followed by 500m Intense (Repeat)*

## HILL TRAINING

This session includes a moderate 1 mile walk to the training hill and is designed to help the athlete obtain some hill resilience so that they will not be phased when encountering hills on the race itself without losing too much speed.

During the hill session the participants will do a series of 200m walks up a fairly steep hill as fast as possible before walking moderately back to the start point.

*6 x 200m means complete 6 sets of the hill.  8 x 200m means 8 times etc.*

## CROSS TRAINING SESSION

These sessions is known by the Mercian Nordic Walking client base as "Trek Fit" and is CV conditioning mixed with a selection of whole body exercises that support the Nordic walking action and promote a whole body approach.

A sample session would include:

*Warm Up*

*4 x 100m high intensity walk sprints with 1 minute rest between. (RPE 8)*

*Press Ups/Chest Band Work*

*45 Degree Angle Pull Ups/Band Work*

*Squats*

*Walk Lunges*

*1600m Moderate paced walk around the track*

*Ankle stability of a wobble board*

The coach will work with individual athletes during these sessions to make sure they are getting their RPE met – See RPE explanation late in this plan.

*If you are not working with a coach then you will need to research an appropriate full body cross training session.*

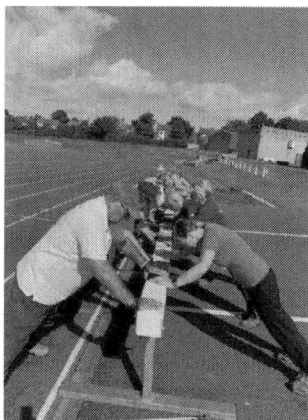

## TECHNIQUE SESSION

As considerable assistance can be achieved from using the nordic walking poles it is advised that you source a reputable instructor so that your technique is of a high standard.

Many instructors offer video technique sessions and these are invaluable.

## REST DAYS

The rest day is to allow the athlete to recover from the sessions.  It will also give the participant time to evaluate their sessions so far.

Participants do not need to take complete rest unless there is a medical reason.  A gentle recreational walk or relaxed swim is perfectly acceptable.

# Programme - Week 1

<u>MONDAY</u>

Baseline Testing

<u>TUESDAY</u>

5km Moderate Intensity Walk

<u>WEDNESDAY</u>

Cross Training Session

<u>THURSDAY</u>

Rest Day

<u>FRIDAY</u>

Cross Training Session

<u>SATURDAY</u>

Technique Session

<u>SUNDAY</u>

7km Moderate Paced Walk

# Programme - Week 2

<u>MONDAY</u>

Cross training session

<u>TUESDAY</u>

7km Moderate Intensity Walk

<u>WEDNESDAY</u>

Hill Session

<u>THURSDAY</u>

Rest Day

<u>FRIDAY</u>

Cross Training Session

<u>SATURDAY</u>

Rest Day

<u>SUNDAY</u>

8 km Moderate Intensity Walk

# Programme - Week 3

MONDAY

Cross Training Session

TUESDAY

8km Moderate Intensity Walk

WEDNESDAY

Rest Day

THURSDAY

Hill Training Session

FRIDAY

Cross Fit Session

SATURDAY

Rest Day

SUNDAY

9km Moderate Intensity Walk

# Programme - Week 4

<u>MONDAY</u>

Cross Training Session

*The second cross training session this week is replaced with a 1600m time trial in order that the participants can see their improvements. The other sessions will remain the same.*

<u>TUESDAY</u>

8km Moderate Intensity Walk

<u>WEDNESDAY</u>

Rest Day

<u>THURSDAY</u>

1600m Time Trial

<u>FRIDAY</u>

Rest Day

<u>SATURDAY</u>

Hill Session 8 x 200m

<u>SUNDAY</u>

10km Moderate Intensity Walk

# Programme - Week 5

MONDAY

Cross Training Session

TUESDAY

8km Moderate Intensity Walk

WEDNESDAY

Hill Session 8 x 200m

THURSDAY

Rest Day

FRIDAY

8km CV Conditioning Session

SATURDAY

Rest Day

SUNDAY

12km Moderate Intensity Walk

# Programme - Week 6

MONDAY

Cross Training Session

TUESDAY

10km Moderate Intensity Walk

WEDNESDAY

Hill Session 10 x 200m

THURSDAY

Rest Day

FRIDAY

8km CV Conditioning Session

SATURDAY

Rest Day

SUNDAY

10km CV Conditioning Session

# Programme - Week 7

MONDAY

Cross Training Session

TUESDAY

8KM Moderate Intensity Walk

WEDNESDAY

5KM CV Conditioning Session (RPE 7/8 for whole walk)

THURSDAY

Rest Day

FRIDAY

8km Moderate Intensity Walk

SATURDAY

Rest Day

SUNDAY

8km CV Conditioning Walk

# Programme - Week 8

An extra day of rest is built into week 8 as athletes near the competition date.

*In the context of sports, tapering refers to the practice of reducing exercise in the days just before an important competition. Tapering is customary in many endurance sports, such as long-distance running and swimming. For many athletes, a significant period of tapering is essential for optimal performance. The tapering period frequently lasts as much as a week or more. This tapering means gradually reducing the exercise over a short period of time then stopping completely when leading up to competitions.- Source Wikipedia*

MONDAY

Rest Day

TUESDAY

6km Moderate Intensity Walk

WEDNESDAY

Rest Day

THURSDAY

6km Moderate Intensity Walk

FRIDAY

Rest Day

SATURDAY

Rest Day

<u>SUNDAY</u>

10km RACE DAY

# The Race

On race day it is suggested that you go for a 1km walk before the race begins. This will serve as a warm up and help to ensure you start the race in the aerobic zone.

> ➢ Arrive in plenty of time.
> ➢ Check your poles and paws.
> ➢ Make sure you have some hydration.
> ➢ Above all else - enjoy the day.

Usually there will be markers counting the race down (9km, 8km etc). To complete the race in 90 minutes you will be walking at a pace of 9 minute/km. So if the conditions are flat then see if you can walk a little bit faster than that pace to "get some time in the bank" for when you hit some hills. Simply set your watch as you pass a marker and aim to be at the next marker at the 9 minute point.

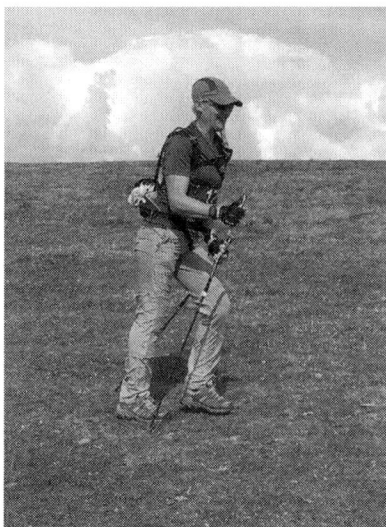

# Final Thoughts

I hope you have enjoyed this training programme.

If you have followed it fully you will be prepared for your race.

Once you have done this challenge then you might consider a half marathon or even a full marathon.

I can be reached at merciannordicwalking@yahoo.co.uk if you wish to get in touch.

Please leave a review on Amazon.

Printed in Great Britain
by Amazon